Birdshot Chorioretinopathy (BSCR)

Birdshot Chorioretinopathy (BSCR)

Frances Foster, MS, NP
Zihan Yu
C. Stephen Foster, MD, FACS, FACR

ISBN: 978-1-7332376-9-7

Eye Words to Know

Autoimmune: An autoimmune disease is a condition in which your immune system mistakenly attacks your body and releases proteins called autoantibodies to attack healthy cells.

Retinopathy: Retinopathy is any damage to the retina of the eyes, which may cause vision impairment. Retinopathy often refers to retinal vascular disease, damage to the retina caused by abnormal blood flow.

Birdshot chorioretinopathy (BSCR): is an eye condition in which painless, light-colored spots develop on the retina. These spots are scattered in a "birdshot" pattern. The cause of BSCR is currently unknown, but it is suspected to be an autoimmune disease.

WHAT IS BSCR?

Birdshot chorioretinopathy, commonly referred to simply as "birdshot", is a rare form of posterior uveitis which mainly affects the retina and choroid. The disease occurs in women more often than men, typically caucasian, and it predominantly affects people in middle age. Given its rarity, patients often encounter delays in diagnosis leading to delays in adequate treatment, and thus risking significant visual loss. "Birdshot" can be a severe and blinding disease if unrecognized or undertreated. If treated properly, it can be cured.

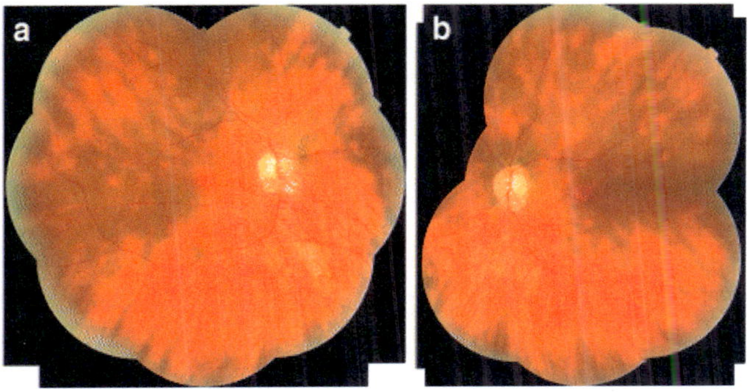

Fig.1 Fundus photomontage of right (a) and left (b) eyes of a patient with BCR revealing both classic creamy ovoid lesions and the linear streaks of more advanced lesions.

What causes BSCR?

The etiology of the disease is, as yet, unknown. There is a class of genes known as human leukocyte antigens (HLA), and specifically one called HLA-A29 (also HLA-A29.2 or HLA-A*2902), that is present in the overwhelming majority of "birdshot" patients, and is thought to be involved in the development of the disease.

Infection, by virus or bacteria, in susceptible individuals is thought to act as a trigger, with the disease then being self-propagated by an autoimmune mechanism.

What are BSCR symptoms?

It is normally a chronic problem, with symptoms that develop and progressively worsen over several months to years.

Early in its presentation, patients may report a range of visual symptoms, the seriousness of which may not be recognized, particularly as visual acuity (VA) is often preserved.

The most common complaints are:

- Floaters and flashes
- Blurry or hazy vision, sometimes described as looking through murky water
- Decreased color and/or night vision
- Glare, photophobia,
- Reduced peripheral vision
- Decreased depth perception

Patients usually do not complain of pain or redness, though it can be present. There are not any systemic diseases that are typically associated with "birdshot".

The disease is bilateral and commonly symmetric, early in its presentation, patients may report a range of visual symptoms, the seriousness of which may not be recognized, particularly as visual acuity (VA) is often preserved. Please pay close attention to your symptoms!

How is BSCR Diagnosed?

A large array of clinical testing can be very helpful, starting with a careful clinical assessment (history, examination and investigations as needed) to exclude infection and systemic disease. In patients presenting with a typical clinical appearance of BSCR, one would order a **blood workup,** especially for the presence of the HLA-A29 gene.

Color vision testing can show mild to severe deficit. Fundus auto-fluorescence may reveal abnormal areas of hypopigmentation that correspond to "birdshot lesions" or overlap areas or normal appearing retina.

Fluorescein angiography (FA) may show window defects in areas of "birdshot lesions" or evidence of macular edema, retinal vasculitis, optic nerve inflammation, or choroidal neovascularization.

Indocyanine green angiography (ICG) is used to evaluate the choroid, and can show hypolucent lesions that are not be visible on dilated exam.

Visual field testing with a blue- on-yellow protocol (shortwave automated perimetry, or SWAP) is more sensitive than normal white-on-white visual field testing, and may show more advanced field defects.

Optical coherence tomography (OCT) can reveal macular edema or epiretinal membranes.

Standard electroretinogram (ERG) can be a very useful tool in both the diagnosis of "birdshot", and in assessing response to therapy, particularly the 30-Hertz photopic protocol, which will often show delayed implicit times and decreased signal amplitudes that may improve with treatment. For some conditions, the passage of time may also help identify the underlying disease.

CAN "BIRDSHOT" BE TREATED?
AND
HOW TO TREAT INFLAMMATION FROM "BIRDSHOT"?

Yes, this disease is very treatable, and after proper treatment, it is even possible to achieve long-term remission of active inflammation while off all medications. The mainstay of treatment in BSCR is steroid-sparing immunomodulatory therapy (IMT).

Immunomodulatory Therapy (IMT)

Immunomodulatory therapy is the standard of care for treating birdshot retinochoroidopathy. The research, by the Dr. C. Stephen Foster, world renown ophthalmologist for ocular inflammatory disease and Founder of OIUF, in treating patients with "birdshot" have shown the most effective initial treatment strategy involves starting combination therapy with mycophenolate mofetil (CellCept®), an anti-metabolite, and modified cyclosporine A, a calcineurin-inhibitor.

In cases of intolerance or poor efficacy, mycophenolate is sometimes replaced with another antimetabolite, or the patient is transitioned to intravenous therapy with a TNF-α inhibitor such as infliximab (Remicade® preferred) or injectable adalimumab with preferred Humira®. Stubborn and poorly controlled disease on these medications may require use of an alkylating agent.

Corticosteroids

Our research has found that patients who have received oral corticosteroids have shown a higher rate of disease recurrence, even after achieving long-term remission on immunomodulatory therapy. Injection into the eye (intravitreal injection) was not shown to have this risk. Topical eye drops are not effective in treating inflammation in the back of the eye.

Corticosteroid Implant

A corticosteroid implant surgically placed within the eye, fluocinolone (Retisert®) and others, can be used for patients who are not able to achieve remission on or tolerate immunomodulatory therapy, or in cases where this option presents less of a burden on life than long-term medical therapy.

What is the length of treatment of BSCR, *and* the maintenance testing?

The combination of cyclosporine and mycophenolate mofetil as well as other immunomodulatory (IMT) regimens were explored in efforts aimed at induction of a durable remission off IMT and no recurrence of BSCR inflammatory activity. It was discovered that if the patient has been in remission, on immunomodulatory therapy, and off steroids for two years or more—depending on the case—we can then consider weaning immunomodulatory therapy for durable remission off IMT.

During treatment, the weaning process, and post-treatment, patients are carefully monitored for reappearance of symptoms or objective evidence of inflammation. The maintenance testing includes ERG, FA, ICG, OCT, blue on yellow visual fields and Snellen VA—all of which serve as indicators of objective disease activity in BSCR patients.

Depending on stage of treatment or remission, maintenance testing for disease activity may be every 3, 6, or 12 months. After several years, durable remission testing can extend from one to every two years.

WHAT ARE THE OTHER PROBLEMS ASSOCIATED WITH "BIRDSHOT", *AND* HOW ARE THEY TREATED?

Cataracts and Glaucoma

Cataracts and glaucoma can both occur as a result of active inflammation or long-term treatment with corticosteroids.

- Cataracts can be removed, ideally when inflammation has been treated and the eye is quiet, but may need to be removed to see and treat problems inside the eye.
- Glaucoma is initially treated with eye drops, followed by laser therapy, and lastly surgery if necessary.

Retina

Problems with the central retina, especially macular edema and epiretinal membranes, are frequently seen.

- Macular edema may resolve when inflammation is treated, however if it persists, it can also be treated with topical NSAIDs (nonsteroidal anti-inflammatory drugs), oral acetazolamide, Intraocular injection of either corticosteroid or a VEG-F inhibitor, and other forms of treatment pending case.

- Epiretinal membranes can be surgically removed if they are felt to cause progressively worsening vision. Intraocular injection of either corticosteroid or a VEG-F inhibitor is extremely effective in treating macular edema. These can also be used to treat choroidal neovascularization, new blood vessels that grow between retina and choroid as a result of a break in the barrier that lies between them.

References

1. Foster, C.S., Birdshot Retinochoroidopathy. Retrieved from https://uveitis.org/patient_ articles/birdshot-retinochoroidopathy/

2. Shah KH, Levinson RD, Yu F, Goldhardt R, Gordon LK, Gonzales CR, Heckenlively JR, Kappel PJ, Holland GN. Birdshot chorioretinopathy. *Surv Ophthalmol.* 2005;50(6):519–41.

3. Birdshot chorioretinopathy: current knowledge and new concepts in pathophysiology, diagnosis, monitoring and treatment: *Orphanet Journal of Rare Diseases.* (n.d.). Retrieved from https://rdcu.be/bU40a.

4. Kiss, Szilard, Muna Ahmed, Erik Letko, and C Stephen Foster. "Long-Term Follow-up of Patients with Birdshot Retinochoroidopathy Treat- ed with Corticosteroid-Sparing Systemic Immunomodulatory Therapy," June 2005.

5. Gasch AT, Smith JA, Whitcup SM. Birdshot Retinochoroidopathy. *Br J Ophthalmol.* 1999;83: 241–9.

6. Rothova A, Berendschot TT, Probst K, van Kooij B, Baarsma GS. Birdshot chorioretinopathy: long term manifestations and visual prognosis. *Ophthalmology.* 2004;111(5):954–9.

OIUF

THE OCULAR IMMUNOLOGY AND UVEITIS FOUNDATION

Dedicated to Eye Disease Cure and Education

The Ocular Immunology and Uveitis Foundation is a 501c(3), not-for-profit, tax-exempt organization. Our mission is to find cures for ocular inflammatory diseases, to correct the worldwide deficit of properly trained ocular immunologists, and to provide education and emotional support for those patients afflicted with ocular inflammatory disease.

We Believe…

- In this day and age, no patients should suffer with poor treatment for ocular inflammatory disease.
- A cure is possible for ocular inflammatory disease.
- We can correct the deficit of properly trained ocular immunologists.
- Patients should have ample support during this time of need.

www.uveitis.org

Notes

Made in the USA
Monee, IL
05 November 2026

67374691R00017